Hear4Life™

How to ACHIEVE BETTER HEARING and IMPROVE YOUR RELATIONSHIPS with the people you love

CHRISTOPHER M. SUMER, NBC-HIS

To my wife Kiera,

for your unwavering love and support; without you I would
not be who I am today. I love, honor, and respect you.
Thank you for being my wife and my best friend.

To my mentor Randy Rose,

for starting me on this journey and providing support and advice.
I also thank you for instilling in me early on that every person
I did not help was "bleeding in the streets." Without your continued
support, I would not be as successful in business as I am.

CONTENTS

Hear4Life™

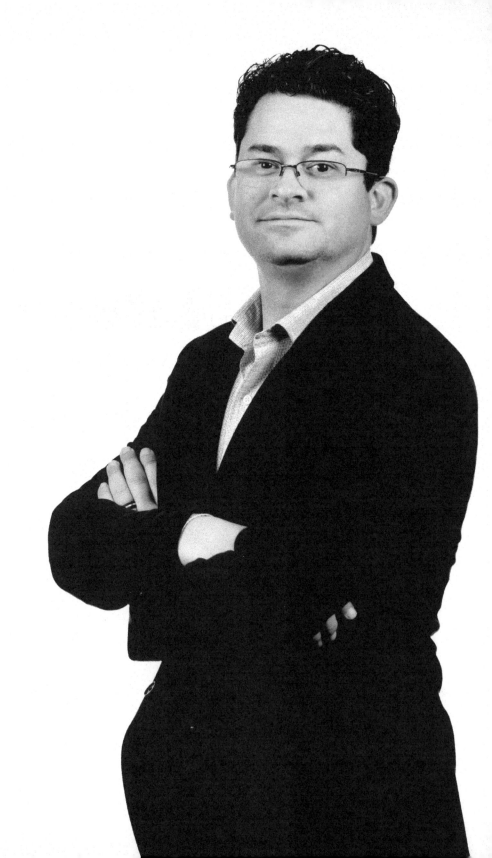

ABOUT THE AUTHOR

Giving the Gift of Sound

I have a passion for helping those with hearing loss reconnect to their hobbies and relationships through the gift of sound.

As a second-generation hearing care professional, my uncle was a hearing care professional, and I used to ride along with him during school vacations. Later, as an adult, I shadowed him while I trained, and it left a lasting impression on me. One day, an older woman accompanied by her neurosurgeon husband came in for a fitting. This woman had never worn hearing aids before, and when she wore them for the first time her whole face lit up, and she started crying. After her husband started talking, she started crying even harder.

I've been hooked ever since.

It is my fervent hope to guide you or a loved one to better hearing.

Christopher M. Sumer, NBC-HIS

Nationally Board Certified in Hearing Instrument Sciences
Director of Operations and Research at Coastal Hearing Aid Center
Assistant Director of HearShare Foundation
Board Member at International Hearing Society State and Federal Advocacy

WHY I WROTE THIS BOOK

It's Time for a Hearing Revolution

With over 48 million Americans suffering from hearing loss, my goal is to help as many people as possible hear well again.

I am so sure I can improve your hearing that I guarantee my work 100%. (Most of my colleagues offer only a 60-or 90-day guarantee.)

But to achieve the best hearing for everyone, there must be a change in mindset for hearing care professionals and the people we serve.

Better hearing isn't about purchasing hearing devices; it's about investing in your communicative ability.

I repeat—better hearing isn't about purchasing hearing devices; it's about investing in your communicative ability. It's about being able to hear your grandkids, going to the symphony, listening to a lecture at a museum, or being able to communicate with family during the holidays without having to turn up the volume on your hearing device.

But too often when I want to suggest the right type of equipment, I am limited by what insurance covers.

I knew there must be a better way, so I created a program to transform the way hearing care is provided that I call Hear4Life, which you can read about in the upcoming pages.

This handbook is a practical how-to guide to find the right hearing care professional who can help improve your hearing. You'll discover loads of actionable items, such as a checklist of questions to ask and tips on navigating finances.

I hope you can find the right professional who can really make a difference in your hearing.

INTRODUCTION

You Are Not Alone

As a matter of fact, you're like most Americans:

- Twenty-five percent of those aged 65 to 74 experience hearing loss.[1]

- Fifty percent of those who are 75 and older have disabling hearing loss.[1]

- And of those, less than one in three wear hearing aids.[1]

But here's the scary thing:

- Three out of five older Americans with hearing loss do not use hearing aids.

- And six out of seven middle-aged Americans with hearing loss do not use hearing aids.

There's a lot more at stake here than vanity when it comes to not wearing hearing aids.

You could be missing out on crucial conversations at work. You could start to feel isolated from your family and friends. More importantly, your mental health could begin to suffer.

There's a strong correlation between hearing health and mental health. According to a report from Johns Hopkins Medical Center, even a mild hearing loss can increase the risk of dementia by 200%, and with severe hearing loss, the rate increases to 500%.[2]

Doctors tell us that treating hearing loss is the best way to prevent it from causing mental health issues, including dementia. In this book, we're going to learn about the link between hearing health and mental health, and we'll walk you step by step through the process of finding a hearing care professional, testing, and financing your hearing aids.

Here's to your health!

Are you missing out on hearing health?

25% of Americans between *65 and 74 years of age* experience hearing loss

50% of Americans *75 years of age and older* experience hearing loss

And of those, fewer than **1** in **3** wear hearing aids

SECTION 1

Busting Five Myths
About Hearing Loss

As a hearing care professional, I see new people almost every day. After they get fitted and wear their hearing aids for the first time, the first thing they often tell me is, "I should have done this a long time ago."

People have so many misconceptions about hearing aids: they're ugly, they're hard to adjust, they're expensive, they don't work, they aren't covered by insurance, they really don't help. Yes, maybe that applies to the big, clunky ones you may remember your grandparents wearing in the 1980s, but lucky you—there's new technology.

As technology has progressed, so has our understanding of the science of treating hearing loss. Hearing loss is closely tied to mental and physical health. The effort we spend on improving hearing pays off in helping prevent cognitive loss and mental deterioration.

These aren't your grandfather's hearing aids anymore.

With so much at stake, why do people put off treating their hearing loss? The following are five reasons I hear almost every week in my practice. Do any sound familiar to you?

Myth #1: I can just deal with it.

It takes time for people to come in for their first visit. For a while, they just don't want to admit that their hearing is decreasing. They have to ask people to repeat themselves. The TV volume goes up just a notch higher. "Why does this generation insist on mumbling?" they may ask themselves.

Hearing loss may be so gradual you might not even notice the rate of decline. But at some point, you must admit that you do not hear as well as you used to. You may be tired of asking family and friends to repeat themselves. So finally, you decide to take the advice of your spouse, kids, or coworkers and make an appointment to see a hearing care professional.

On average, it takes people seven years before they come in for a hearing appointment.

Yes, on average, it takes people seven years before they come in for a hearing appointment. But why wait? The earlier you come in, the better your chances are for preventing permanent loss. Some people even say they're too old to get hearing aids. "I only have a few years left, anyway," is something I hear quite often. I remember meeting Glen, a World War II veteran. He was a nice guy who walked into my office with his cane at

103 years old! He said, "let's see what you can do!" And sure enough, I was able to help improve his hearing again.

Meeting Glen really changed my thought process. Age has nothing to do with it. After all, even if you have just a few years left, don't you want as much connection as possible?

So, I invite you to make an appointment. While we can't cure progressive degenerative hearing loss, we can lessen its impact. We can provide you with the most opportunities to help you retain as much of your hearing as possible, stimulate the brain, and reduce the possibility of hearing-loss–induced dementia.

Myth # 2: I'll have to deal with salesmen trying to rip me off.

Marketers love promoting to seniors because they know seniors will spend money on their health. As a result, the medical industrial complex has evolved to sell you everything from medicine to glasses, and yes, hearing devices.

But when it's time to treat your hearing, you should never feel like someone is selling you something. I strongly recommend that you seek out a certified hearing care professional. Ask your friends (and their parents) for recommendations. Or read reviews on Yelp, Google, and Facebook. I passionately suggest that you work with a licensed hearing care professional with an office, not a salesperson working out of a big box retailer. Your specialist will work with you to find the best treatment.

> ## You need to approach treating your hearing loss with the same seriousness as any other medical condition.

Don't forget that your hearing loss is a medical condition, and you need to treat it with the same seriousness as any other medical condition. Only a trained hearing care professional is certified to determine the proper course of treatment for your hearing loss.

Myth #3: The insurance process is too confusing.

Yes, I hear you. Whether you have private insurance, Medicaid, Medicare, or a combination of the three, navigating medical insurance isn't always easy.

But luckily, over the past two or three decades, hearing has been given higher priority. In fact, most plans consider an annual hearing checkup by a certified professional as preventative care and will pay for 100% of the cost. Plus, more insurance plans will pay for part or all the costs of hearing aids.

If you need help with your insurance company, the patient care coordinators in your hearing care professional's office will be knowledgeable about the health plans in your area. They should be able to assist you with the process of getting reimbursed by your insurance company.

Most insurance plans will cover anywhere from 10% to 100% of the cost of hearing aids.

If your insurance only pays for part of your hearing aids, your specialist's office can work with you to come up with a financing plan to pay the difference.

Myth #4: Hearing aids are too expensive.

You probably know someone who has paid thousands of dollars for hearing aids, only to not wear them. Some devices are made only to amplify sound—your dinner companions in a restaurant, the waiter walking by, the clinking of dishes being washed in the kitchen. The cacophony of noise makes it hard to hold a conversation.

Other hearing aid shoppers may have purchased theirs at expensive stores that claim to carry premium devices. What they really paid for is high rent in a fancy mall. Hearing aids aren't fashion accessories, so there's no need to pay more for a trendy brand name. You want to invest your precious funds in hearing aids, not high rent.

I encourage you to work with licensed hearing care professionals. They will have your best interests at heart and won't try to sell you what you don't need. Quality hearing care professionals will offer devices at a variety of price points to fit your budget. They can work with your insurance company to get some or maybe even all the costs of your hearing aids covered. However, if it turns out that you have to pay most of the out-of-pocket costs, your hearing care professional should be able to offer you several financing options so you can extend payments for a few months to a year or so.

What is the real cost in quality of life if you don't treat your hearing loss?

The most important question you should be asking is what is the real cost in quality of life if you don't receive the treatment you need for your hearing loss? Are your relationships becoming strained because you are missing out on conversations? Do you avoid going to restaurants and other public places because the environments make it difficult to understand people? Is your hearing loss playing a factor in your performance on the job? What sort of cognitive abilities are being lost because your mind must overcompensate for not hearing everything? Are you increasing your chances of dementia?

Due to improvements in medicine, we're living longer than ever. But with increasing life spans, the occurrence of dementia is expected to triple over the next thirty years. Our bodies can often remain healthy longer than our minds. Caring for our loved ones with dementia can be expensive, running into tens of thousands of dollars per year. But studies are now showing that addressing hearing loss is the most modifiable risk factor of developing dementia.

Myth #5: I'm too young to wear hearing aids.

Yes, those old banana hearing aids your grandfather wore were ugly and hard to adjust, and they didn't work very well. Yes, you are too young to wear hearing aids like that, because hearing aids have improved.

Hearing aids are now so small, people will barely know you're wearing them. The devices are high-tech wonders and super adjustable, so they'll conform to what's comfortable for you. But still, I understand if you aren't thrilled about attaching a technical device to your body all the time to treat a medical condition.

Whether you have two months, two years, or two decades left, don't you want the highest quality of life possible?

For some people, wearing a hearing aid screams out "I'm old. I'm old. I'm old!" Others ask, "I'm not going to be here much longer, so why should I wear a hearing aid?" My answer is, "don't you want to enjoy your remaining days with your loved ones by your side? Don't you want to be able to talk to them and understand what they're saying? Whether you have two months, two years, or two decades left, don't you want the highest quality of life possible?"

Because really, nothing says "old" like constantly asking people to repeat things. And nothing can transform you into a grumpy old person faster than self-imposed isolation because you are too embarrassed to wear a hearing aid.

MYTH	TRUTH
I can deal with it.	The earlier you get treatment, the earlier you can reduce cognitive overload (stress on the brain).
I don't want to deal with salesmen trying to rip me off.	You can work with a hearing care professional dedicated to improving your hearing, not meeting a sales quota.
The insurance process is too confusing.	The office of a good hearing care professional should have customer care specialists who will advocate for you with your insurance company.
Hearing aids are too expensive.	The real question to ask—what is the real cost in quality of life and relationships if you can't hear your loved ones, friends and co-workers.
I'm too young to wear hearing aids.	New hearing technology is so small, people won't even notice you're wearing anything.

Hearing again after 30 years

"I was told I would never hear from my left ear due to nerve damage. After visiting Chris and his wonderful staff, I am hearing from my left ear for the first time in over 30 years. His techniques and devices are a miracle, and I would recommend Coastal Hearing to anyone."

Janet J.

SECTION 2
How Hearing Health Is Linked to Mental Health

You picked up this book because you or a loved one is at the point where you are considering hearing aids. Before I share how to find a hearing care professional or about the hearing aid fitting, let's dive into the connection between hearing health and mental health.

Hearing loss can cause mental degradation.

There are different types of loss. Conductive hearing loss occurs when sound cannot pass into the inner ear, and it's often caused by wax build-up, infection, or injury. A hearing care professional can identify this type of loss and is often easily corrected.

Sensorineural hearing loss is caused by problems with the inner ear's acoustic nerve pathways. The inner ear, known as the cochlea, contains nerve endings that are responsible for translating incoming sound information through electrical signals. When the cochlear cells die or become damaged, the nerve pathways to the brain are also damaged.

Hearing degradation can occur very slowly, translating to decreased cognitive function in areas including speech, language, hearing, and memory.

A study conducted by researchers from Johns Hopkins University School of Medicine and the National Institute on Aging suggests seniors with hearing loss are significantly more likely to develop dementia over time.[1]

A lot of people ignore hearing loss because it's such a slow and insidious process as we age.

Frank Lin, MD, PhD
Johns Hopkins University School of Medicine

The researchers found that subjects who had hearing loss at the beginning of the study were significantly more likely to have developed dementia by the end of the study. Compared with volunteers with normal hearing, those with mild, moderate, and severe hearing loss were 200%, 300%, and 500%, respectively, more likely to develop dementia.

HEARING LOSS LEVEL	INCREASED CHANCE OF DEVELOPING DEMENTIA
None	0%
Mild	200%
Moderate	300%
Severe	500%

So, when the loss of hearing occurs slowly and is at first hard to detect, corresponding mental degradation may also occur.

"A lot of people ignore hearing loss because it's such a slow and insidious process as we age," says study leader Frank Lin, MD, PhD, assistant professor in the Division of Otology at Johns Hopkins University School of Medicine. "Even if people feel as if they are not affected, we're showing that it may well be a more serious problem."[2]

Hearing loss contributes to three major causes of dementia: social isolation, change in brain structure, and cognitive overload. I'll take you through each one and give pointers on how to deal with each symptom.

Social Isolation: When You Feel Alone

Social isolation is often the first symptom when someone experiences hearing impairment. If people with any type of hearing loss cannot hear the conversations around them, their conversations tend to become more limited in number. They might hear parts of conversations and then ask questions that are out of context, making them feel awkward. As a result, they become even more hesitant to take part in conversations.

To compound matters, when people with hearing loss stop communicating with others, they start to experience even more isolation, and this can exacerbate any other mental health problems they might suffer from.

Hearing Loss ➜ Social Isolation ➜ Cognitive Impairment

Hearing loss can reshape a person's social environment, alter relationships and cause a shift of responsibilities. If a person is hard of hearing, he or she may delegate tasks to his or her partner—such as answering the door or telephone—or may rely on the partner to repeat everything. The person might also turn up the volume on the TV or radio, which can annoy family members, roommates, or people living below or next door.

Hearing loss can reshape a person's social environment.

The way people cope with their hearing loss may also further isolate them. They might avoid situations out of fear of potential embarrassment or because they know they can't control the unpredictable environment of a public space.

Because hearing loss can happen at an almost imperceptible rate, people might adjust their behavior very slowly until the culmination of the small adjustments suddenly becomes noticeable. For example, casual acquaintances might interpret behavior as rude or a sign of boredom when it's really a lack of engagement. When people are asked to frequently repeat themselves, they may avoid talking to a person with hearing loss.

People with hearing loss often feel frustrated by their difficulties in communicating with others. They might be embarrassed to ask others to repeat themselves. These feelings of frustration can evolve into depression if they're not taken care of.

A study of 2,300 seniors over the age of 50 conducted by the National Council on Aging (NCOA) found that those with hearing impairments were more likely to experience depression or anxiety, and they were also less likely to engage in social activities, which can further exacerbate their social isolation.[4]

WHAT YOU CAN DO
Help Prevent Social Isolation

Transportation Issues	If you can't drive anymore, ask a family member or friend to pick you up. Chances are, one of your friends would be happy to drive you. Many cities also offer dial-a-ride services to seniors.
Regularly Scheduled Events	Weekly scheduled events keep seniors engaged and give them something to look forward to. Is there a senior group at church? Can you volunteer at the library? Join a garden club? Seeing people regularly can do a lot to lift your spirits.
Share a Meal	Family dinners were once a daily highlight. Scheduling a regular lunch or dinner date once a week or even once a month helps to maintain ties to families and friends.
Care for Another	Maybe it's a pet. Maybe it's a plant. But caring for somebody or something else can help reduce feelings of isolation.

Hearing loss speeds up brain shrinkage.

As people age, their brains shrink a little—it's a natural part of the aging process. But for individuals who are experiencing hearing loss, that shrinkage can happen at an even faster rate.

Another study by researchers from Johns Hopkins University and the National Institute on Aging found that hearing loss seems to accelerate brain shrinkage. Accelerated brain tissue loss can manifest as dementia, falls, and diminished physical and mental health.

Previous studies comparing the brain structures of people with hearing impairments to those with more normal levels of hearing revealed that the brain structure responsible for processing sound tended to be smaller in the hearing-impaired individuals. However, Dr. Lin, the lead researcher, says they don't know whether those brain structure changes happened before or after hearing loss.

Accelerated brain tissue loss can manifest as dementia, falls, and diminished physical and mental health.

The scientists also reported that people with hearing loss lost more than an additional cubic centimeter of brain tissue every year compared to those with normal hearing. Specifically, shrinkage occurred in the part of the brain responsible for processing sound and speech. It is possible these areas could have shrinkage or atrophy due to lack of stimulation, but no part of the brain works in isolation. The middle and inferior temporal gyri also play key roles in memory processing and sensory integration and have been shown to be involved in the early stages of mild cognitive impairment and Alzheimer's disease.

"If you want to address hearing loss well," study leader Dr. Frank Lin continues, "you want to do it sooner rather than later. If hearing loss is potentially contributing to these differences we're seeing on MRI, you want to treat it before these brain structural changes take place."[3]

What's my suggestion? Don't delay getting your hearing checked!

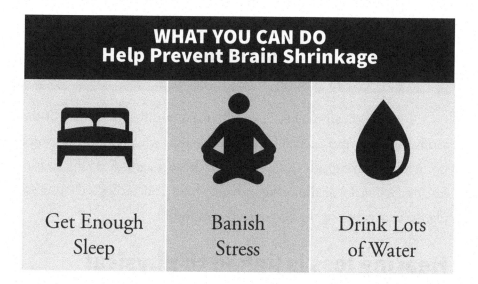

**WHAT YOU CAN DO
Help Prevent Brain Shrinkage**

Get Enough Sleep | Banish Stress | Drink Lots of Water

Cognitive overload means the brain is working too hard.

When you don't hear entire parts of a conversation, your mind has to work extra hard to figure out what was said in the previous sentence. Meanwhile, the speaker has moved on to new information for you to process. This can take a huge amount of energy, leading to exhaustion and causing what is known as cognitive overload.

When you add in the challenge of a noisy background, the stress level can rise even further. Retreating to a quiet room may give you a break. If you're at work, you can record important conversations (with permission) and then transcribe the audio so you can make sure you don't miss important details.

Your mind has to work extra hard to figure out what was said in the previous sentence.

Of course, hearing aids can really make a difference. State-of-the-art hearing aids can reduce background noises while amplifying voices (something hearing aids couldn't do two decades ago). A skillful hearing care professional will also make sure your brain is neurologically processing the conversations the hearing aid is capturing.

Hearing loss is linked to physical health.

Older adults with hearing loss are more likely to be hospitalized and to experience times of inactivity and depression. In fact, they are 32% more likely to have been admitted to a hospital than those with normal hearing.[5]

"Hearing loss may have a profoundly detrimental effect on older people's physical and mental well-being," says Dr. Lin.

Older adults with hearing loss are more likely to be hospitalized and to experience times of inactivity and depression.

Balance is centered in people's ears, and sound plays an important role. If you can't hear well, you're more likely to fall. Data from the 2001–2004 National Health and Nutritional Examination Survey revealed hearing loss is a significant factor in falling over. A mild hearing loss is associated with nearly three times the likelihood of falling.

A French study[6] also revealed that people with untreated hearing loss were 28% more likely to have an accident while bathing or dressing and 13% more likely to experience hazard risk when using the telephone, managing money, shopping, or during transport. People who wore hearing aids had no increased risk during these activities.

"Our results underscore why hearing loss should not be considered an inconsequential part of aging but an important issue for public health," says Dr. Lin.

Our results underscore why hearing loss should not be considered an inconsequential part of aging but an important issue for public health."

Frank Lin, MD, PhD, assistant professor in the Division of Otology at Johns Hopkins University School of Medicine

WHAT YOU CAN DO
Healthy Aging

Exercise	Commit to an aerobics/exercise plan. Try going for a 30-minute walk every day or ride an exercise bike. Swimming and water aerobics are low-impact cardio options. Try tai chi and yoga (even chair yoga) help reduce stress.
Learn a New Hobby	Explore some new interests.
Read	If you love to read, keep on reading. If you need some encouragement, join a book club.
Take a Class	Go back to school or take a class at your local senior center.

The early treatment of hearing loss is the single most effective modifiable factor in the prevention of dementia.

Don't delay getting your hearing checked.

As you've read, the consequences of untreated hearing loss can be detrimental to you and your family. But taking care of it early has a host of benefits, including increased brain function, decreased isolation, a lower risk of dementia, and improved physical and mental health.

SECTION 3

Selecting A Hearing Care Professional Who's Right For You

Maybe you've had this conversation recently play in your head:

"I wonder if it's time to get my hearing checked. Nah, I'm doing just fine."

This conversation might even repeat for a few years.

But if your spouse or child is asking you to get a hearing test, it might be time for you to do it. If you're not able to fully participate in conversations, you can be missing out on a vital part of maintaining deeper relationships with your loved ones. Conversations with your loved ones are too precious, and life is too short to be left out of them. The American Medical Association recommends people 50 years and older to get their hearing tested.

Over 48 million people suffer from hearing loss. Of those age 70 and older who could benefit from wearing hearing aids, fewer than 30 percent have ever used them.[1]

Of those who are

70 and older

who could benefit

from hearing aids,

only **1** in **3**

wear hearing aids

Maybe it's time to see a hearing care professional.

Below are some points to consider when you're deciding if you need to see a hearing care professional and, if so, what to look out for to find the right specialist to help you.

Asking People To Repeat Themselves

Do you find yourself asking your friends, family, and coworkers to repeat themselves? In particular, the softer voices of women and children may be harder to understand. It can sound like everyone's voices are muffled.

Noisy Places Make Conversation Difficult

Has going out to dinner with your children and grandchildren lost its appeal because the background noises drown out the conversation? Maybe you have started to stay home because you can't hear people when you're in a restaurant, at a party, in church, or attending family events. However, if you don't engage in conversation, you're more likely to feel detached, even if you're surrounded by your loved ones.

Blasting The TV Loudly

Do your next-door neighbors know what you're watching on TV? When you begin to experience hearing loss, you're more likely to increase the volume on your TV or radio to try to hear. This is a sign that it's time to get your hearing checked.

Ringing In Your Ears

Ringing in your ears isn't just a figure of speech—it's a real medical condition known as tinnitus. Ringing in your ears can occur after exposure to very loud noises. If the ringing persists, it's time for a hearing test.

Missing The Sounds Of Daily Life

Most attention is given to not being able to hear people speak, but don't forget about the sounds of everyday life. Can you hear the sounds on the crosswalk at a busy intersection? Can you hear your cat meow? Do you sleep through your alarm? Hearing keeps you connected to your environment and helps keep you safe.

Talking On The Phone Is Hard

You might not have any trouble talking face-to-face but holding a conversation on the phone may be difficult. At work, you may be missing out on vital information about projects and talking on the phone may be the most important way you keep in touch with distant loved ones.

Don't shortchange these relationships. Instead, take a hearing test so you can get treatment for your condition. You will need to make an appointment with a hearing care professional to evaluate your treatment needs.

Maybe it's time to get your hearing checked if you:

✔ are always asking people to repeat themselves

✔ have trouble hearing conversations in noisy places

✔ turn up the TV volume

✔ experience ringing in your ears

✔ sleep through the alarm

✔ find talking on the phone is difficult

What's a hearing care professional?

Hearing care professionals are experts who have undergone training to learn how to test hearing, fit hearing aids, and offer follow-up services. Once a hearing care professional is licensed by the state, they can work in private practice, for public agencies such as the Veterans Administration and Medicaid, in manufacturer-owned stores, and for large retailers that might sell everything from hearing aids to automotive oil to five-pound boxes of Cheerios.

How to select a hearing care professional.

The best way is to ask for referrals from friends, coworkers, and family members. Once you have a list of names, here are some things to look for and some questions to ask when considering which one is best to help you.

❶ Do they offer case studies?

A hearing care professional should be able to share case studies of people they have helped. They should be able to tell you how a person's life had been affected by hearing loss and how hearing aids improved their life. You should also be able to find case studies of people with hearing problems like the ones you face.

❷ Do they have an office?

I strongly suggest going to a hearing care professional at their own of-fice—first, because they should have their credentials and affiliations displayed, and second, because the fact that they have an office means they are more likely to have all the equipment to conduct the tests you need. While it's true that some hearing care professionals who are associated with large retailers such as Costco and Walmart may offer lower prices, their service and follow-up may be lacking. Sometimes it takes a third or fourth visit to optimize a hearing aid for the best performance. In addition, going to a manufacturer's store will mean you're limited to options provided only by that manufacturer. I believe that going to an independent hearing care professional is your best option to enjoy a premier experience and have the widest selection to choose from.

❸ Are they concerned with your brain?

Of course, a hearing care professional is concerned with your hearing, but they should also focus on your brain too. Hearing health involves more than just the ability to amplify sound. It's also about improving the connection between your ears and your mind.

❹ Are you charged a fee for your first visit?

Most companies will not hire someone without a job interview first. Likewise, your first visit should be a complimentary consultation where you and the hearing care professional get to know each other first. This gives you the opportunity to ask the questions I am reviewing here and to inquire about the process and the hearing aid devices. This isn't just a transaction to purchase hearing devices. You are also counting on the professional knowledge and service of this hearing care professional to optimize your device for your needs.

❺ Is there a guarantee for products and services?

Purchasing hearing aids is an investment of both time and money. Therefore, you want to have the assurance that your hearing care professional will stand behind their treatment and the devices they suggest for you. You need to ask:

- Do they have a risk-free guarantee, so you won't be stuck with ineffective treatment?
- Do they offer additional adjustments so the device can be optimized?
- Do they offer follow-up care to ensure your treatment continues to be effective?

We offer a **100% guarantee** that you'll hear better or **we'll refund your** money.

❻ Have they kept up to date on technology and treatment?

Hearing aid technology has improved by leaps and bounds in the last few years. Hearing technology nowadays is more precise and much smaller than in the past—most people won't even notice you're wearing hearing aids. A new technology called NeuroTechnology™ places the device in your ear canal to make it almost undetectable.

❼ Is the price of supplies included?

Hearing aids require you to change filters and tips periodically. Are these supplies included in your contract, or are they an additional cost? Be clear before you sign and ask what the prices will be for additional supplies to avoid any financial surprises later.

❽ How many follow-up appointments are included?

Once you receive your hearing aids, you can count on needing a period of adjustment. Your hearing care professional will need to optimize your device to your needs. You might notice an improvement in some situations but still look for more in other situations. Some hearing care professionals offer these follow-up appointments for free, while others charge for them. It's your responsibility to ask before you sign any contract.

❾ Do they offer personalized service?

You want a hearing care professional who has the experience of serving hundreds or even thousands of people throughout their career. But when you're getting fit for hearing aids, you want them to understand this is your first time and that you need them to take the time to explain things to you and adjust to fit your needs. This can do a lot to reduce any anxiety you have about the process.

⑩ What do other customers say about this hearing care professional?

Almost every hearing care professional should have numerous reviews on forums such as Yelp, Google, and Facebook. You can also ask your hearing care professional for referrals you could talk to about their services.

Questions to ask when visiting a hearing care professional:

1. Do they offer case studies?

2. Do they have an office?

3. Are they concerned with your brain?

4. Are you charged a fee for your first visit?

5. Is there a guarantee for products and services?

6. Have they kept up to date on technology and treatment?

7. Is the price of supplies included?

8. How many follow-up appointments are included?

9. Do they offer personalized service?

10. What do other customers say about this hearing care professional?

What Is Tinnitus?

Maybe you hear the sound of the ocean. Or hissing, whistling, whooshing, or clicking.

This could be tinnitus. Otherwise known as ringing in your ears.

Tinnitus is a way your ears are telling you that something is wrong with them. Usually it is caused by damage to or loss of sensory hair cells in the inner ear (cochlea).

The whooshing or ringing sounds tend to be more noticeable at night when life's distractions are at a minimum. Tinnitus is a symptom of greater ear problems. There is no cure, but it can be managed.

What's in a name?

Tinnitus is derived from Latin, meaning "to ring or tinkle."
There are two ways to pronounce the word. (And both are correct!)

ti-NIGHT-us
typically used by patients and laypeople

TINN-a-tus
typically used by clinicians and researchers

The Causes of Tinnitus

Exposure to Loud Noises

Did you attend a lot of concerts as a kid or play in a band? Do you listen to loud music on your headphones for hours a day? Do you work on a construction site or at an airport? Loud noise can destroy delicate hair cells in the inner ear. This can cause permanent damage because the hair cells don't grow back.

The March of Time

As you get older, age-related hearing loss, known as presbycusis, occurs at higher frequencies.

Earwax Buildup

Wax can accumulate in the ear canal and cause tinnitus. Sometimes, if you can have the wax removed, the symptoms of tinnitus disappear.

Meniere's Disease

This is a disorder of the inner ear that can cause hearing and balance problems. People who suffer from it may feel pressure in the ear.

Ototoxic Drugs[2]

- non-steroidal anti-inflammatory drugs (NSAIDs)
- certain antibiotics
- certain cancer medications
- water pills and diuretics

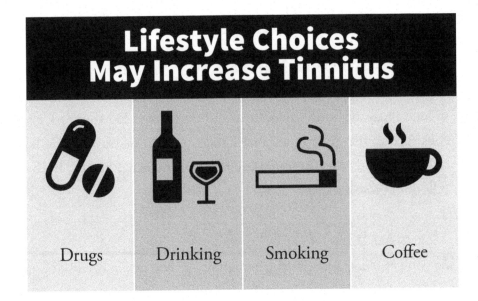

Ways You Can Manage Tinnitus

Create your own white noise.

Use a fan or air conditioner to create background noise at night to help you sleep.

Play soothing music.

Music will help your brain focus on something besides the ringing.

No caffeine!

Say good-bye to coffee, soda, energy drinks, and all of your other favorite caffeinated beverages. Caffeine increases blood pressure, which can aggravate your tinnitus.

Stop smoking. Now.

Smoking inhibits blood flow to the sensitive nerve cells that control hearing.

Explore acupuncture.

Some people have reported relief with acupuncture and other alternative medical approaches.

Loud noise? Hello earplugs.

If you're going to be mowing the lawn or operating a power saw, earplugs help reduce ear damage.

Ways Your Hearing Care Professional Can Manage Tinnitus

There is no proven cure for tinnitus, but your hearing care professional can offer treatment that could help reduce the impact of the ringing in your ears. While treatment won't completely erase the effects of tinnitus, some of these treatments can help reduce the emotional and cognitive impacts of this condition.

Hearing Aids

Hearing aids can amplify environmental sounds. While the ringing may still be heard, it will be partially masked by ambient sounds. This allows your brain to focus on something besides the consistent ringing in your ears.

Sound Therapy

Sound therapy uses external sounds to alter a person's reaction to tinnitus. A single-function device, such as a radio, an app on a smartphone, an electric fan, or a fountain, can provide masking noises to camouflage the ringing sounds. The most effective noise should create positive responses for each person and encourage the brain to focus on something besides the tinnitus.

Modified sounds or notched music devices offer modified music or algorithmically- generated sounds in specific frequencies to expressly address your tinnitus. These devices are not worn all the time but just at select times, such as during therapy sessions or before bed.

Cochlear Implants

Cochlear implants are surgically implanted devices that restore the sensation of sound to deaf people. The sound amplification may help combat the effects of tinnitus. Cochlear implants work on the same principle as hearing aids—they increase outside sound stimulation, helping to distract the brain from the perceived sounds of tinnitus. Cochlear implants are only helpful to people who are deaf in both ears. Make an appointment with an otolaryngologist to see if you're a good candidate.

Behavioral Therapy

Behavioral therapies are among the most effective treatments for tinnitus. By reducing anxiety and stress, behavioral therapies address the emotional toll of tinnitus. It's important to recognize that while the condition itself isn't debilitating, one's reaction to tinnitus can make it almost impossible to live with, so the goal of behavior therapy is to reduce your negative reactions to the symptoms of tinnitus.

A behavioral therapist can offer you coping mechanisms to help reduce your brain's attention to your tinnitus.

Behavior therapies can be delivered in group settings or one-on-one settings. The overall goal is to increase pleasant activities and learn relaxation techniques and skills that help reduce the negative thinking associated with tinnitus.

Drug Therapies for Tinnitus

Unfortunately, there is no pill you can take to cure tinnitus. However, some drug therapies can reduce the effects of the condition.

Antidepressants and Anti-anxiety Drugs

These drugs don't directly address the tinnitus condition itself but rather the stress and anxiety that can be related to tinnitus. These drugs help break the cycle of tinnitus > anxiety > tinnitus worsens > more anxiety.

Common antidepressants prescribed for tinnitus include:

- Clomipramine (Anafranil)
- Desipramine (Norpramin)
- Imipramine (Tofranil)
- Nortriptyline (Pamelor)
- Protriptyline (Vivactil)

Commonly used anti-anxiety medications include:

- Alprazolam (Xanax)
- Clonazepam (Klonopin)
- Diazepam (Valium)
- Lorazepam (Ativan)

Medications That Should Be Avoided

Some people have tried taking over-the-counter medications, including antihistamines, anticonvulsants, anesthetics, and even anti-alcohol drugs, to deal with their tinnitus, but these medications have not been proven to improve the tinnitus condition. You should also shy away from any "miracle cures," because there simply are no drug cures for tinnitus at this time, though there is robust research in the development of such medications.

You can overcome tinnitus.

"I have struggled with Tinnitus for one year. I have had four nose/ear/throat doctors tell me there was nothing they could do to help me with it. Each time I got that verdict, I felt scared, defeated, and hopeless. Also, the daily and nightly noise in my head was becoming unbearable.

One day I was doing my work of researching this illness online when I found Coastal Hearing Aid Center in Encinitas. Everyone here was so kind and supportive of my illness and gave me hope that one day I would have a solution for it. That very day after a complete hearing test, I was handed a pair of hearing aids! I cried! For the first time in ten years the noise was gone in my head! These were special hearing aids, just for retraining, and helping to tamp down the noise. And it works! Please if you have tinnitus, don't wait! Get down here, get checked and get your life back!"

Carmen K.

SECTION 4
Your Hearing Test

4

Everyone has their own unique journey of hearing loss. So, I have built a process that allows me to treat you in a personal and educational environment where I can offer personalized treatment and customized hearing and cognitive training solutions. Because technology is always evolving, I am constantly upgrading my testing process to achieve the most precise results.

The Initial Consult

The first consultation (which is free) will allow us to get to know one another. The first question I am going to ask you is, "why are you here?" Our conversation will be like peeling back the layers of an onion and discovering where you're coming from. Recently, one gentleman came to see me at the urging of his wife. I asked him if he went to restaurants anymore, and if not, why. The results from his exam confirmed everything he said, and that really opened our conversation. He became more engaged as I started to talk about available options.

I'll also ask if you have any concerns or fears about the process, and I'll answer any questions you may have. Most people come into their initial consultations with their arms crossed. What are you trying to sell me?

is what they're often thinking, even if they don't say it out loud. If they don't want my help and a family member dragged them there, I will give them the information and the answers they are looking for and invite them to call me when they're ready to receive my help.

I never want to twist someone's arm to go through hearing treatment. I would much rather provide information and then wait until they are comfortable with treatment. I want everyone to have a positive experience. As long as they agree they are going against good advice, we can shake hands and part as friends.

You're getting more than your hearing treated—you're getting treated as a whole person. We will ensure that we do all the necessary work to keep you best connected with your loved ones and friends.

Questions I will ask:

- Why are you here?
- Have you had your hearing checked elsewhere? What was your experience?
- What comments have your family, friends, and coworkers made about your hearing?
- Is there a family history of hearing loss?
- Have you been exposed to excessive noise through work, accidents, or concerts?

You'll want to come to the initial consult prepared with questions. (For starters, check out the list of questions at the end of the previous section.) You might also want to bring your spouse, your adult child, or a friend with you to the appointment—not only for moral support but also as a second pair of ears. You might be so overwhelmed or nervous that you forget to ask certain questions or forget the answers you receive. So, bring a list of written questions, and while you're here, feel free to take notes as you receive answers.

I'll also provide a short presentation on how to treat hearing loss. Everyone's treatment is a little different because everyone's hearing is a little different.

The Discovery

Before we begin treatment, you'll need to undergo a battery of exams to hone in on every aspect of your hearing, from your ear canal all the way to your brain.

Otoscopy (ear canal check)

Your hearing care professional will check the canal for excess wax (medically known as cerumen). The best practices can show you the landmark of your ear canal using video otoscopy. A tiny camera will be inserted into your ear canal to ensure a healthy and clear external ear.

Tympanometry (middle ear analysis)

This checks your eardrum and the section behind it where the middle ear bones—the hammer, anvil, and stirrup (the malleus, incus, and stapes)—are found.

The Beep Test (air and bone conduction test)

You probably remember this test from school: "Raise your hand when you hear a beep." This test checks your ability to hear tones of different pitches in each ear. Soft foam earphones, inserted into your ear canals, deliver a series of tones in the ears. You will press a button or raise your hand when you hear the tone. This test indicates if your hearing is caused by a problem in the middle ear or inner ear.

Cognitive Hearing Test (how well you understand words)

How well do you understand what's being said? This test's results, also known as "Word Discrimination Scores/Ability," help determine how well you hear language and process conversation. You'll be asked to repeat a set of words at a conversational level. People with normal hearing usually catch between 96% and 100% of what's being said, while people with mild to moderate hearing loss will understand about 50% to 60% of what is being said. This is to establish a baseline for levels of hearing.

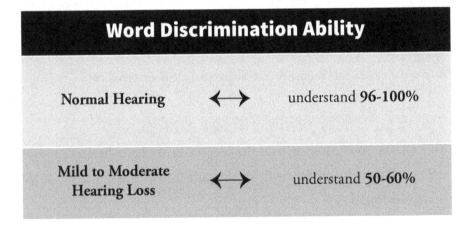

Word Discrimination Ability

Normal Hearing ⟷ understand **96-100%**

Mild to Moderate Hearing Loss ⟷ understand **50-60%**

Then you'll repeat this test, except this time the volume and clarity will be optimized to address your hearing loss. This second test will provide your "Hearing Potential Score," and the results should capture what you are capable of hearing with a device that is optimized for your condition.

For example, if you previously achieved 50% to 60%, you could now score 90% or greater.

Cognitive Hearing Test With Background Noise

Not being able to hear a conversation with background noise is the first warning sign of hearing loss, so it's very important that your ability to understand language with background noise is quantified. The test for this is called the "Quick Speech in Noise Test" (QuickSIN), which gauges your difficulty in understanding and following conversations in environments with background noise.

During the test, sentences are played, and we ask you to repeat them. With each new sentence, the background noise becomes louder and louder by increments of five decibels.

Individuals with normal hearing can hear almost every single word at every iteration of the test; however, people with hearing loss experience significant difficulty as the background noise gets louder than 10 decibels.

The Review

All your test results will be compiled in an audiogram, which is sort of like a report card for your hearing that we will review with you. This audiogram notes your hearing loss in frequencies and decibels and reports the type, pattern, and degree of your hearing loss as well as the percentage of normal conversational speech that you are still able to hear.

When we review all the tests, we will sit down with you and your loved ones and discuss the results of the tests to allow you to understand the results, as it is important for you to understand the extent of your hearing loss. It is also important for your family and friends with normal hearing to understand the extent of your hearing loss. This will help them better understand what you are going through.

We will then relate these results to your concerns about your hearing, and we will discuss what your options are. We will take the time to find out your preferences so we can take them into account when coming up with a hearing plan for you.

Getting Fitted With Your Hearing Devices

Selection of Technology

After your initial hearing tests and feedback, we'll figure out the best products, or system that would help you hear the best you possibly can. Our decision is based on the best technology that's available. Some manufacturers offer products designed for long-term users while devices are best for transitional users. Sometimes I may suggest accessories like remote microphones or a TV streamer in addition to your hearing devices.

Molds are Made

Before we make molds of your ears for your hearing devices, I'll look inside to make sure your ear canal is clear of debris or foreign objects which could drastically improve your hearing. Then I'll insert cotton to protect your ear drum. I'll inject a two-part silicone (vinyl polysiloxane) into your canal to make a reverse cast. Then the mold is sent to a lab that builds your hearing device.

Follow up Fittings

Once your hearing devices are received from the lab, I'll fit them and check that they are not uncomfortable. Then we'll test the sound you receive. I'll start you at a comfortable listening level and may adjust your levels over the course of a couple of visits.

Annual Evaluation

I'll test your hearing every year because your hearing loss and cognitive ability can change without you being aware. By addressing changes early, I can help you avoid greater hearing loss.

The journey starts today.

After we gather your medical history and past experiences, perform otoscopy, tympanometry, air and bone conduction, and cognition assessments, we will discuss all the findings and how they relate to your everyday life. We can begin your journey to better hearing quality by treating your impairment as soon as day one. Research has proven that early intervention with hearing loss has profound cognitive benefits that begin as early as 14 days after starting treatment.

"I was so totally pleased and happy I had given Chris a try. He is not only knowledgeable, but he truly cared about solving my problems and gave me something that solved all my issues—clarity, no background noise interference, total comfort.

I had no idea my hearing was so poor until I could actually hear everything being said around me and on the tv or radio."

Toni R.

NeuroTechnology™ —because we hear with our minds as well as our ears.

The problem with old-school hearing aids.

Hearing aids do just what their name promises: they aid hearing by amplifying the sounds around you. The problem is that hearing aids amplify not only the sounds of conversations with your loved ones but also the sounds of the kitchen clatter in the restaurant and the fifty other conversations around you. The result: old-school hearing aids work well in one-on-one conversations in quiet places but not so well in noisy environments.

The traditional approach to this problem has been directional microphones. For example, if you were wearing old-school hearing aids in a restaurant and the noisy kitchen was to your right, you could press a button to turn on a directional microphone. The problem was that you would hear nothing in other directions, including any people sitting on your left or right.

NeuroTechnology™ does more than amplify sound.

NeuroTechnology™ improves auditory input to the brain.

Hearing health involves more than your ears. NeuroTechnology™ is a term for top-tier technology that offers a more sophisticated approach than traditional hearing aids by simulating complex patterns to help replace diminished auditory input to the brain. The result? You'll be able to hear in all situations, even in restaurants with your family.

NeuroTechnology™ is a technology, not a brand or manufacturer. We select the technology that will work best for you.

How NeuroTechnology™ works:

- **Improved Clarity**—NeuroTechnology™ restores clarity for hard-to-understand parts of speech such as 'sh,' 't,' and 's'. Soft-speech boosters enhance clarity across the entire spectrum of speech.

- **Increased Surround Sound**—NeuroTechnology™ helps create a more natural listening experience by pinpointing sound in all directions, enabling listeners to enjoy a clearer auditory experience. Old-school hearing aids don't offer auditory clues about depth and height. With NeuroTechnology™, taking a walk in the park or going to dinner with friends is a far more enjoyable experience.

- **Noise Cancellation**—People with hearing loss have a terrible time distinguishing conversation from background noises. NeuroTechnology™ offers noise cancellation that enhances speech while reducing background noise by up to ten times.

NeuroTechnology™ is almost invisible.

NeuroTechnology™ uses tiny state-of-the-art technology that makes our hearing aids very discreet. It's so lightweight you won't even remember you're wearing it.

NeuroTechnology™ hearing aids fit well because they:

- fit deeply inside your ear canal for perfect comfort and invisibility
- easily adapt to changing environments and provide automatic volume control
- provide wireless streaming to your smartphone to keep you connected to your TV, music, and media
- enhance the sounds of conversation while minimizing distortion of loud noises

NeuroTechnology™ enhances brain function.

NeuroTechnology™ uses microtechnology to support working memory, selective attention, and processing speed. It can analyze the auditory environment in real time and enhance speech and reduce distortion caused by loud noises.

(*The Hearing Review,* Dr. Desjardin, University of Texas, El Paso)

Experience improved hearing with NeuroTechnology™

30% **increase in speech comprehension**	Advanced technology separates speech from background noise by up to 10dB.
20% **increase in mental recall**	Increased clarity enhances the brain's ability to remember what was said.
20% **reduction in hearing effort**	Less effort is required by seniors to hear in noisy environments.

Bluetooth transforms NeuroTechnology™ into smart technology by enabling:

Hands-free wireless hearing on the phone

Low battery reminders by ear, phone, text, or email

Wireless compatibility with TV

Control of internet-connected devices at home

Living With Your NeuroTechnology™

While NeuroTechnology™ is the next generation in hearing devices, there are some things you can do to prolong the life of your new device.

- **Don't sleep with your NeuroTechnology™**—Sleeping with the devices in can cause discomfort. It is easy for the devices to fall out of your ear canals if you toss and turn at night, making it easy to lose them. And you will wear out your batteries twice as fast.

- **Don't go swimming in your NeuroTechnology™**—Unlike old-school hearing aids, NeuroTechnology™ is water resistant and is rated to survive being immersed up to three feet in water. Still, we advise you not to shower or swim in your new hearing devices in order to preserve them!

Caring For Your NeuroTechnology™

Yes, you must clean your hearing devices. Use a lint-free cloth to wipe down the unit every day to prevent buildup of dead skin cells, earwax and dust from building up in the microphones. (You should receive these with your NeuroTechnology™. You should also change out the wax filters and domes (which hold the device in place) and microphone filters (if your unit has that capability).

Grace & Granville

"My husband, Granville, and I met when we were both older. Granville had already been wearing hearing aids for years.

Granville was born in England and originally developed hearing problems after serving as a pilot with the Royal Air Force in WWII. During the war, he went to Lancaster, California, for training and fell in love with California. He talked about visiting Hollywood during leave and having people buy him drinks and spotting movie stars. After the war, he moved to California and became a U.S. citizen.

Over the years, his hearing got bad, and he was deaf without the hearing aids. His insurance network would only cover a few brands, and none of them made a difference. We would drive to get them adjusted once or twice a week. Finally, his audiologist said, "We can't do anything more."

Finally, our dentist (of all people) suggested that we pay out of network and go see Chris at Coastal Hearing Aid Center.

Chris took his time with Granville and outfitted him with the most powerful hearing aids available. He made new molds for Granville so they would be tight fitting but still comfortable.

At age 96, Granville got NeuroTechnology™ and was able to hear everything, even when he was in a crowd. When he went to the hospital, he could hear what the doctors were saying. He was able to talk on the phone once again with his 90-year-old brother, who still lives in England. And now we can go to eat with another couple and Granville can easily partake in the conversation. And he was able to watch his favorite musical once again— Kiss Me Kate, starring Howard Keel.

After seeing Granville's success, I thought I should give hearing aids another try. I had tried them previously, and they were awful and so uncomfortable. Chris did a wonderful job helping me, and now I hear better than ever. Chris is so knowledgeable about different types of hearing aids and can find the right one for you.

I haven't had any problems, and they are so comfortable. I can't believe I waited so long."

Grace

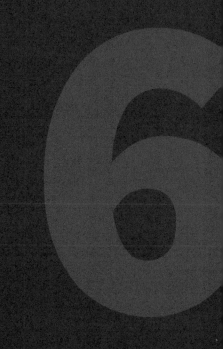

How To Pay For Your NeuroTechnology™

Why do people put off getting hearing aids? One of the biggest reasons is cost. Without even knowing the price tag, many people avoid getting their hearing checked for years.

Don't let this happen to you. Chances are your insurance company will pay for a hearing test and part or all of your hearing aids. While we're not accountants, we do work with people all the time to find ways to finance their NeuroTechnology™. Chances are we've worked with your medical insurance company.

Flexible Spending: Pay For Your Hearing Devices and Enjoy Tax Savings

It might take a little planning to take advantage of a flex spending plan if one is available to you through your job or your spouse's work. A flex spending plan lets you put aside a certain amount of tax-free income per year to be used for medical expenses. (And yes, NeuroTechnology™ and any other hearing devices are medical expenses.)

Here's how to make flex spending work for you:

- **Plan Ahead**—Most employers only let you sign up for flex spending at the start of the year, but you can usually sign up if your circumstances change, including marriage, divorce, job loss, or loss of spouse's insurance.

- **Know Your Amounts**—Be sure to know what limit your employer sets. It also doesn't hurt to have a rough idea of how much your hearing devices may cost, so go ahead and schedule your initial consultation. You don't want to put too much into your account because most accounts have a policy of "use it or lose it" during the calendar year. (If you do have some extra funds at the end of the year, you can always stock up on supplies.)

Financing your NeuroTechnology™

Maybe your insurance company will cover only part of the cost of your NeuroTechnology™. If that's the case, you might not have funds available to pay the entire price of new hearing devices. Financing the rest may be your best option. Our office works directly with a bank to help finance low-rate loans so you can get your hearing treated the right way. We all want to avoid debt, but if there's been one consistent theme in this book, it's this: **Don't put off treating your hearing loss.**

Irreparable damage can happen. The sooner you treat it, the less permanent damage will occur.

Someone I now work with first went to Costco looking for hearing aids. They offered her a $900 device, which was beyond her budget. She called me asking if there was some miracle that could happen. I contacted a bank that I regularly work with, and we came up with a creative payment plan that was affordable for her and her husband. She received top-tier technology, and now she can hear again.

Most hearing care professionals should be able to help with financing. Look for common options such as:

- 0% interest for 12 to 18 months
- 12.9% interest with monthly payments locked in for 3–5 years
- direct-finance plans that may offer even lower terms

How To Work With Your Insurance Company

Healthcare is always changing—what your plan will cover can easily change from year to year. While our billing specialists are familiar with almost every local insurance policy, we still check every policy because conditions can vary among individuals.

But the good news is that most insurance plans—and Medicare—will pay for the cost of a hearing test. And most insurance plans will cover at least part of the cost of hearing treatment.

Take these steps to get clear answers from your insurance company:

① Call your insurance company and ask if they cover hearing treatment.

② Don't hesitate to call your insurance company several times. You'll be surprised at the variety of answers you receive. (Tip: always get the name of the employee you speak with and a reference number to document the conversation.)

③ Rely on the patient care coordinators most hearing care professionals have in their offices. The patient care coordinators are used to working with insurance companies, and they'll advocate for your right to have coverage for hearing health.

HearShare Foundation

I got into this business to improve the hearing of people who need it. I never, ever want to turn someone away because they can't afford the hearing devices they need for their best hearing. I try to be as creative as possible to make things happen.

I started collecting hearing aids from people who had passed away or upgraded to better technology in order to give them to someone in need, so my wife and I started the HearShare Foundation, a 501(c)(3) nonprofit organization which provides reconditioned hearing aids as they become available. There is an application process for this top-end technology. We have also worked directly with major manufacturers to obtain new hearing aids.

Here's one example of how we've been able to help:

An elderly woman needed hearing aids, but all her finances were tied up in a court case. Her daughter approached us looking for reconditioned hearing aids. I was able to work with a manufacturer to provide top-end hearing aids. She can hear everyone talk again. This has been a transformative experience because now she can hear the judge during her legal case proceedings.

Hear4Life™

A revolution in hearing treatment that puts you, not the insurance companies, first.

I go to work every day with a mission—to provide the gift of better hearing to as many people as possible. I have extensive knowledge of hearing products and can often suggest the technology that will enable people to hear well again.

But too often, I have found myself hindered and limited by insurance companies in terms of what brands they would approve—which often weren't what the people I'm caring for really needed. I knew there had to be a better way to provide premier hearing care.

So, I asked myself what the perfect hearing health program would look like. As a result, I developed the Hear4Life™ membership, a program designed to provide you with 100% guaranteed hearing care, something unprecedented in the hearing care industry.

A flat monthly fee gives me the flexibility to switch between products when I am not getting the results for you that I think are possible. This lets me make the determination—not the insurance company. If I think cognitive training would help, we'll add it into your routine. If we need to add remote microphone at a particular frequency, we can. We can change equipment or other streaming accessories to provide better hearing as often as we need to.

Please accept my 100% guarantee that I can improve your results. If you're not satisfied, you will receive a refund and we'll part as friends.

A Simple Flat Inclusive Rate

This inclusive rate covers everything you need for better hearing (excluding surgery).

- **New Hearing Devices As Often As You Need Them—** If your hearing changes, we'll change out your hearing aids as needed.

- **All Adjustments Included—**See us as often as you need to.

- **100% Guarantee—**Most of my colleagues only guarantee their work for 45 to 60 days. We are proud to offer a 100% guarantee. (We're serious about improving your hearing.)

- **Brain Training (Brain HQ™)—**Because even the best hearing aids are simply tools, we address your cognitive decline as well.

- ***You* Call The Shots, Not Your Insurance Company—** We aren't beholden to any brand or technology. We will suggest the technology we believe will work best for you. If we need to try another brand, we can.

- **Priority Treatment—**If you need an emergency adjustment, I will be available for you. No waiting around over a long holiday weekend.

Frequently Asked Questions

If I have hearing loss, won't my regular doctor tell me?

No. Most general practitioners don't regularly check for hearing loss. And in the quiet setting of a clinic, your hearing may be fine compared to a noisy restaurant or gathering.

I can still hear. Do I really need to have my hearing tested?

Yes. Changes in your hearing can be very subtle, so you won't notice them. But the earlier you treat hearing loss, the more you can prevent permanent damage to your hearing.

What should I look for in a hearing care professional?

First, make sure your hearing care professional is licensed, which means they have received extensive training in hearing loss treatment. Second, check their references and testimonials to make sure that they provide quality service.

I tried hearing aids 15 years ago and found them to be very uncomfortable. Have they changed much since then?

Yes. Advances in technology have made hearing devices smaller, more powerful, and more accurate. It's definitely time to recheck your hearing!

What happens at the initial consultation?

The initial consultation gives us an opportunity to meet and for you to ask any questions. If you are ready to proceed, we can also perform your initial hearing tests. These tests give us a baseline against which to measure future improvements in your hearing.

How much will the initial consultation cost me?

The initial consultation is absolutely free. I want you to be comfortable when making the decision about working with me.

What sort of tests do you perform at the initial testing?

I'll perform tests to determine your hearing levels in both quiet and noisy situations. I'll also test to discover what parts of people's speech you tend to miss the most.

How do I get fitted for a hearing aid?

After your tests, we'll review your results and select the products or systems best able to improve your hearing. We will choose the most suitable technology for you; we are not limited to the products of a single manufacturer. Then I will make molds of your ear canals and send the casts out to a lab. The lab will create your hearing device.

Can hearing aids be adjusted?

Yes. In fact, to perfect your hearing, several follow-up visits may be required. It may be best to begin with your hearing devices at a lower level, and then when you are used to them, I can adjust the levels to improve your hearing. Most follow-up adjustments can be performed remotely (TeleHealth) from the comfort of your home and in front of your smart device.

Can I bring a family member to my appointments?

Yes, I think this is a great idea, and I highly suggest it. There is a lot going on when you are getting your hearing tested or adjusted and having another person there will help you remember details about your hearing and the reasons why we chose the treatment we did. It also helps family members to realize the extent of your hearing loss.

How often should I get my hearing checked?

I suggest once a year because your hearing can slowly change over the course of a year. I want to address any loss of hearing quickly, before permanent hearing loss occurs.

How can I pay for my hearing devices?

Several insurers, including Medicare and Medicaid, cover at least part of the cost of hearing devices. Some people are offered flexible spending programs by their employers, or secure low-interest loans. My office works with financial institutions who will offer loans at a very reasonable interest rate.

In an emergency, can I make an after-hours appointment?

Yes. It is rare. If your device malfunctions due to a loose wire, lost domes, or irritation, call my office as soon as you can, and we'll try to take care of it quickly.

Does ringing in my ear mean anything?

The ringing you hear in your ear is called tinnitus. It is usually caused by damage to the inner ear, medically known as the cochlea. Within the cochlea, little hair-like cells have nerves that connect to the brain. When the hair cells are damaged, the connection to the brain is lost. The ringing is your body's way of telling you that something is wrong with your ear. While we might not be able to cure your tinnitus, I can offer ways to reduce its effects.

What is this NeuroTechnology™ that I keep hearing about?

It isn't a brand or a manufacturer; it's a technology.

In the past, hearing devices merely magnified the surrounding sounds. NeuroTechnology™ works on a more sophisticated level. It can improve the clarity of hard-to-understand parts of speech. It improves surround sound and enables a clearer auditory experience. It can also help to cancel out background noises while amplifying conversation.

Can I sleep while wearing my NeuroTechnology™ device?

We encourage you not to, in order to give your ears a break. You'll also run through the batteries twice as fast.

Can I swim while wearing my NeuroTechnology™ device?

While it is rated for both dust and moisture resistance, we still encourage you not to bathe, shower, or swim while wearing your device.

How do I clean my NeuroTechnology™ device?

It's simple. Just take a smooth cloth without lint and a brush to wipe your device. This will help remove oils, wax, and skin cells that can build up. Every month or so you will want to change the wax filters, ear domes, and microphone filters. Keeping your device clean keeps the mess away!

Why did you start Hear4Life™ and how can it help me?

My purpose is to help as many people as possible hear the world around them. Too many times, someone's insurance won't cover the brand of hearing aids, accessories needed, or a service package that can support someone's ongoing needs. Treating hearing loss is something we need to invest in to ensure proper hearing and cognitive health. So, I offer people the choice of paying a flat monthly fee to ensure I will always be able to offer the best devices and services to improve your hearing. We know your NeuroTechnology™ won't last forever; with this program you are guaranteed an upgrade every 48 months or less. You are never stuck with ineffective and outdated equipment that keep you from hearing your best.

Scientific Sources

Introduction

1 https://www.nidcd.nih.gov/health/statistics/quick-statistics-hearing

2 https://www.hopkinsmedicine.org/news/media/releases/hearing_loss_and_dementia_linked_in_study

Section 2

1 https://www.hopkinsmedicine.org/news/media/releases/hearing_loss_and_dementia_linked_in_study

2 https://www.hopkinsmedicine.org/health/conditions-and-diseases/hearing-loss

3 https://www.hopkinsmedicine.org/news/media/releases/hearing_loss_linked_to_accelerated_brain_tissue_loss_

4 https://www.ncoa.org/wp-content/uploads/NCOA-Study-1999.pdf

5 https://www.hopkinsmedicine.org/news/media/releases/hearing_loss_in_older_adults_tied_to_more_hospitalizations_and_poorer_physical_and_mental_health

6 French epidemiological study (The PAQUID Study) of a sample of 3,777 individuals aged 65 or older who had been followed for up to 25 years. The study was led by professor Hélène Amieva. "Death, Depression, Disability and Dementia Associated with Self-Reported Hearing Problems: A 25-Year Study" was published in Journals of Gerontology: Medical Sciences in January 2018. Sources: PubMed and Journals of Gerontology: Medical Sciences

Section 3

1 https://www.nidcd.nih.gov/health/statistics/quick-statistics-hearing

2 Source: ATA.org

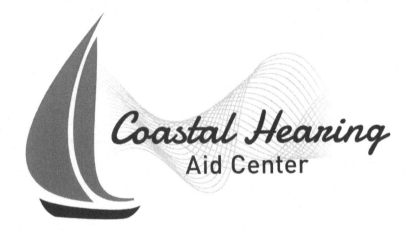

Take the First Step to Better Hearing. Visit

CoastalHAC.com

for a Complementary Consultation.